What's Wrong With My Child?

Struggling with Sensory Integration Dysfunction

By
Shelly R. Wilson

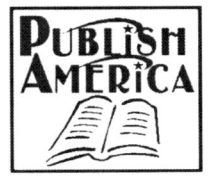

PublishAmerica
Baltimore

© 2006 by Shelly R. Wilson.

All rights reserved. No part of this book may be reproduced, stored in a retrieval system or transmitted in any form or by any means without the prior written permission of the publishers, except by a reviewer who may quote brief passages in a review to be printed in a newspaper, magazine or journal.

First printing

At the specific preference of the author, PublishAmerica allowed this work to remain exactly as the author intended, verbatim, without editorial input.

ISBN: 1-4241-1323-7
PUBLISHED BY PUBLISHAMERICA, LLLP
www.publishamerica.com
Baltimore

Printed in the United States of America

This book is dedicated to my son, John Marcus Wilson.
I love you with all my heart.

This book was not written to embarrass or degrade you. I wrote this book to tell your story of the struggles and triumphs of living with Sensory Integration Dysfunction.

I want parents and children to know that there is always hope.

With love and lots of support, a person living with SI Dysfunction can learn to cope and become a happy and productive adult.

Acknowledgments

There are so many people I need to thank.
First of all I want to thank God, for giving me the patience to help my son.
I also want to thank my husband, Larry for all the support in the world.
Thank you to Megan for helping her brother become the man he is today.
Because of her aggravation, it pushed Marcus to do things he may not have wanted to try.

The following people are special to our family and to Marcus for all their love and support.
Thanks:
JW. And Georgie Wilson
Neill and Wanda Black
To all of our family members
Marcus knows how much his family loves him and we thank you so much.

Marie Matthews, Janet Klements, Elaine Roberts, Angela Williams, Jann Dworsky, Traci Newman, Mary Ann Simpson—teachers
W. D. Bruton, Jim Perkins, Phillip Lowe—band teachers
Peggy Smith—Principal
Nancy Mercer, Elizabeth Geiger—school counselors
Mary Ann Punchard, Karen Wiley Connell—Occupational Therapists
Marc's friends:
Zeb Chambers. Eric Warren, Justin Bulls, Randi McMullen, Rhianan Sliger
Clint Blair, Jimmy Gault, Colt Stewart, Kurt Smalls—Walker

Jesus and Nick Guerrero, Avery Sader,
Mildred Brooks—manager of KB Toys
Patti Granger—Assistant manager of KB Toys
Our Friends:
Paul and Lola, Eric, and Jon Malmin, Laurie Browning
Eddie and Nita Bulls, Kathryn Swanger, Marc and Earl Ann Bumpus,
First Baptist Church family, Troy, Texas

Chapter 1
Baby Days

M"*arcus catch the ball. Come on it won't hurt you. See it's soft."*
As I threw the ball to my 2 year old son, he moved away and did not even attempt to try and catch it. He did not really enjoy playing outside. Marcus would much rather play in the house. I was noticing a lot of things about him that I thought were peculiar.

*****

Marcus didn't enjoy being touched or held very much. I thought that I had learned lot about babies and young children in my twenty six years of living, but this was different. I had always loved babies and I knew how to change diapers and feed them. I thought that was about all there was to taking care of a baby. My sister had twin girls and I had helped her with them when they were little and I thought when I got pregnant, that I was ready. I just didn't know that it could be so hard.

*****

Marcus was born on August 4, 1982, when I was twenty six years old. His father, Larry and I were so happy that words cannot describe the feeling. Marcus was three weeks early. He also weighed only 4lbs. 9ozs. After he was released out into the world through cesarean section in which he was breech, he grew rapidly and everything seemed great.

We lived in a rural part of Arizona at the time and I had none of my family there. I was born and raised in Texas. For the most part I stayed at home, sometimes fourteen hours a day, all alone with my new child, so I observed a lot. My husband, Larry worked long hours building a power plant and we lived over an hour away from the job sight. Most mornings he would leave the house around five a.m. and he would not return until around six or seven p.m.

I was so content with Marcus, that Larry being gone a lot wasn't so bad. Marcus kept me busy and there were other young mothers in the neighborhood that also had new babies. About twice a week we would get together and have lunch. We would exercise, sew, and visit. Most of all, we would play with the babies and swap stories. It made our time go by faster and we were not so lonely. Those days kept me going.

I was really homesick and did not enjoy living in Arizona. I prayed a lot that we would someday be able to move back to Texas and be with our families. I had never been away from my loved ones for so long. I wanted my mother and father to see Marcus and experience his baby years.

Larry was also leading the music at a Baptist Church in our community. We enjoyed the fellowship of the members and it helped having friends in the church. The little old ladies always had advice for me about how to take care of Marcus. I was having trouble burping him and I was afraid he would get sick. One older woman told me to rub his back. I had already tried that and Marcus didn't like it at all. He would try to move away from me and wiggle out of my lap. That was the first thing I remember he did that I thought was odd. I loved to rock him when he was very small and he seemed to enjoy it.

As he got bigger, I remember that he had a lot of ear infections. Some nights I would lay on a pallet in his room on the floor and hold him all night. With a high fever he would cry from the pain. We lived forty miles from the nearest hospital. He took his share of Amoxicillin.

I also began to notice that Marcus did not want to be laid on his stomach. Before he learned to roll over, if I laid him on his stomach he would cry and wiggle around until I turned him over. I thought all babies should sleep on their stomachs so if they spit up, they wouldn't choke. That was 1982, and in those days we didn't know what we know now. Marcus did learn to roll over at about three months old, much to his excitement. Then, every time that I would lay him on his stomach, he would struggle until he rolled over onto his back. He would look at me with triumph and seem to say, " Yea! I did it. Now, leave me alone."

When all the other babies in our mother's group began to crawl, I was frustrated because Marcus wouldn't stay on his stomach long enough to learn. We all bought walkers, so when we were at each other's houses, the babies could see each other and play. We also could feed them in the walkers and not have to have highchairs.

I had always heard that babies should crawl before they walked and I was determined that Marcus *would crawl*. I would sit on the floor with him and lay him on his stomach. Of course he would immediately try to roll over. I would hold him and put him up on his knees and try to show him how to crawl and the battle would be on. He hated that. He would cry and fuss and it was hard not to let him have his way.

Marcus loved being in the walker. By the time he was seven months old, he had that walker mastered. He could go all over the house. One of his favorite things to do was to turn the knobs on the television. We had an old hand-me-down television from Larry's grandmother, and it didn't work very well. I just knew that Marcus was destined to become a TV repair man when he grew up. When I put him in his walker, inevitably he would make a beeline for the TV. I would say, "Marcus, no, no." He would just look me straight in the eye and put his little fingers on the knobs and start turning. If I got up, he would stop and watch me to see what I would do. I would spat his hand and tell him not to play with the knobs and when I turned my back, he would start all over again. *NO, I am not a child abuser*. I did not spat him hard enough to hurt him. I barely touched him. I just wanted to get my point across.

From the time Marcus was born I used a playpen. He had a big square one. I wanted him to be in the room with me most of the time, except at night and I wanted him to get used to it. When he finally did begin to crawl, which took a while, the playpen was a life saver. While I cooked I would put him in the kitchen with his toys and he was happy and safe. When he was playing TV repairman and just wouldn't stop, I could put him in the playpen and give him toys and he was a happy guy.

We also had a big wood stove in the living room. Marcus learned the meaning of "HOT" very early on. That was another good reason for the playpen. I do believe that starting a child in a playpen at birth is a good thing. Both of my children used one and it saved me a lot of worries.

Marc was hooked on a pacifier. All I had to do to get him to sleep was give him the pacifier and either rock him or put him in the bed and he would go right to sleep. Marcus had a favorite stuffed animal. It was a elephant that played, "You are my Sunshine" and it's head would move around while it played. He loved to sleep with it. It wasn't long before the elephant had a broken neck. It was well loved. I noticed as Marcus got older that he really liked all of his stuffed animals and always had a bed full. This was the start to his playacting. I read to Marcus everyday from the time he was born until he could read for himself and even after that. I also sang to him and played music all the time. I wanted him to have a good background in music. We are all very musical and he loves music now.

He talked very early and I guess it's because I talk a lot. I have been known to be called a "motor mouth" before, well maybe more than once. I guess he just picked up on all that talking because he began talking when he was about eight months old. No, he did not recite the *Pledge of Allegiance*, but he did start picking up little words quickly. Of course *"Dada"* was his first word. After all of the hours I spent with that child and his first word was *"Dada"!* His father was so proud, but I was a little disappointed. He did pick up *Mama* soon enough and I thought everything was going along well.

*****

The week before Marc's 1st birthday he finally took his first steps without help. We had been working with him a lot and he did finally learn to crawl, *under duress*. We were so excited because we were going home to Texas for his first birthday. We were flying and I was hoping that he would enjoy the new experience. My family had only seen him once since his birth and I wanted so much to show him off. My younger sister has a son, Luke, only a year older than Marcus and I wanted them to know each other and to be playmates. My sister and I are very close and I hoped they would be also.

A couple of days before we were to leave, Marcus was walking from my chair to the coffee table and he started falling. It was like slow motion. I couldn't catch him. He hit his right cheekbone and he screamed. I picked him up and his cheek was already starting to bruise. I think I cried more than he did. I called a retired doctor in our small community and he said if Marc didn't pass out and if his cheek bone was not sunk in, then he was probably fine. I watched him all day afraid he was badly hurt. Sure enough it was only a bruise. His face healed in a few days.

Around the time that he turned a year old, he decided that he didn't want to be rocked any more. He would go to the refrigerator and beat on the door. He wanted his bottle and wanted to be put to bed. It was strange, but that's what I did. It became a pattern.

There was a very nice park in the town just seventeen miles north of us. On warm Saturdays we would take Marcus to the park and have a picnic. He did not enjoy the playground equipment. He would only get on the smallest rocking horse or the baby swing, but he did not like it. The slide was off limits completely. I just thought he was little and when he got bigger things would change, but he was really afraid of the slide.

When Marcus was sixteen months old we finally sold our house and moved back home to Texas. I was so happy to be back to civilization. We moved into an apartment which was a new experience for all of us. Shortly after moving, Marcus gave up the bottle. I bought some sipper seal cups and he liked drinking out of them.

Chapter 2
Toddler Days

Marcus was still sleeping in his crib and he seemed to feel safe there. He never tried to climb out and when he wanted down he would call me to come get him. We moved back to Texas right before Christmas and my mother gave Marcus a rocking chair. It was very small and all Marcus would have to do was back up and sit down. He wouldn't do it. I would have to pick him up and put him in the chair and when he wanted down, I would put him down. The same thing happened with the couch. Marcus would not climb up or down from the couch by himself.

He was a quiet child and not rowdy at all. He was happy with a book or music. He loved to watch Sesame Street and Mr. Rogers. Marcus never enjoyed playing with toys that other little boys liked. He didn't care to play with cars or trucks. He was scared of a ball and would not even try to catch one.

Luke, Marc's cousin was a rowdy, loud, and active child. He would run through the house and jump on the furniture. He loved to play any kind of ball and loved the outdoors. They were so different. I thought at first it was just the difference in their ages. I thought if we would just give it another year, Marcus would be the same rowdy, loud, regular kid. It didn't happen.

There were other things I began to notice also. His sense of taste started to change. He did not like chocolate at all. He would not eat any meat except chicken or fish. Also he disliked any foods with a tomato product in them. That meant no spaghetti, ketchup, or barbeque. He would eat most vegetables, but Marcus was never a heavy eater. After a few bites he would be finished. After he gave up the bottle, Marc wouldn't drink milk anymore. Finally Nestles began making strawberry and banana flavoring mix and I could get him to drink a little milk with the flavoring mixed in.

While living in the apartments he developed another ear infection and in the middle of the night his eardrum burst. While he was sick all he wanted to eat was Malto Meal. He called it "Macco". I would let him sit on the counter by the stove and help make it. After that, for weeks he would eat nothing but Malto Meal. I told the doctor and he said that it wouldn't hurt him and Marcus eventually began eating normally again. His love for Malto Meal lasted many years to come. In fact in the winter I still make it for him when he's home.

*****

After living in an apartment for six months, we moved to the country to a rent house. It was nice to have our own space again and it was quiet. I'm just not a city girl.

There was a lot of room for Marcus to play and it was quiet.

On August 4, 1984 Marcus turned two years old. He was so cute and we were very happy. We bought him a Big Wheel and he learned to ride it all over the place. It sat low to the ground and he loved it. At first it scared him, but it wasn't long before he was riding by himself. If you remember the Big Wheels, a child didn't have to have balance and it didn't take a lot of coordination to ride. It was a little kid toy.

We also bought Marcus a ball for his birthday, but he wouldn't play with it. I'd say, "Marcus catch the ball. Come on it won't hurt you. See it's soft." As I threw the ball to my 2 year old son, he moved away and did not even attempt to try and catch it. He did not really enjoy playing outside. He would much rather play in the house. I was noticing a lot of things about him that I thought were peculiar.

On August 10th we bought a house in a small town close to our parents. Marcus became so creative. He loved to color and play act. The *Dukes of Hazard* was one of his favorite shows. He had a small Tyke Bike that he rode in the house and when the "Dukes" came on, Marcus would run and jump on the bike and play Dukes of Hazard. I would ask him which Duke he was and he would say, "Dukes of Hazard." I'd say, "No, Marcus, there are two of them. Which one are you?" Once again he'd say, "Dukes of Hazard." I don't think that he understood the question. Marc would not wear shorts in the summer because the Dukes didn't wear shorts. I finally convinced him that the Dukes wore shorts in the summer, but it was winter where they lived. I guess he wasn't looking at Daisy Duke, Ha!

Marcus became more fascinated with books. We read all the time. He seemed to want to learn everything. He was shy with strangers, even my parents. It took him a while to warm up to them. He was definitely a homebody. He was happy staying at home and playing. He wasn't really a bother because he enjoyed playing alone.

*****

One day not long after Marc's second birthday, we planned a trip to my grandmother's house. She was getting pretty old and she loved seeing Marcus. My oldest sister, Leta was going with us. Marcus was still sucking on his pacifier and Leta hated it. I wasn't worried about it. I thought when he was ready to give it up, he would. When we got ready to leave, Marc couldn't find his pacifier. We looked everywhere. We had never lost a pacifier. I was always very organized with his things and I couldn't understand how it could be gone. I accused Leta of getting it and throwing it away. She assured me that she didn't. We left for my grandmother's without it and I told Marc that when we got back we would look for it. He forgot about it until bedtime and then he wanted it. I hadn't bought any more spare ones since he was getting older, but we just could not find it. I told him that we probably dropped it outside and a puppy found it and was sucking on it. He began to laugh. He finally did go to sleep without it and after a few days he learned he could live without it. I will still wonder what happened to it. It is just one of those mysteries that cannot be explained.

*****

Between the ages of two and three he began to watch more television and I noticed that he began acting out the shows. He *became* the characters. He was so cute. I also noticed that he seemed to be a smart child. I worked with him a lot, teaching him his letters and numbers early and I believe Sesame Street helped also. He loved all the characters and I bought him the stuffed animals. He had just about all of them. When Sesame Street came on, Marc would go get all of the animals and line them up on the couch, and when each character came on, he would act out the scenes.

Marc loved commercials and he would always sing along. When he was two years old, something really funny happened. I was teaching him his letters and when we got to the letter M, Marcus said, *"Cratase."* At least that's what it sounded like. I would repeat that the letter was a M, but he would say, "NO, *Cratase*." Boy, I was so confused. The child's name began with a M and he called it a *Cratase*. All of the other letters he pronounced correctly. I gave up on the M and frankly I just forgot about it. I couldn't win. One day as Larry and I were going down the highway we passed a "McDonald's" restaurant. Marc sang, "*Cratase*, oh McDonald's." I then realized what he was saying. I asked Larry if he had heard what Marcus had just said. There was a McDonald's commercial on television at that time, that said, "*Great taste* oh, McDonald's." Marcus thought the M was the golden arches and then it made sense. My child wasn't crazy and neither were we. It all made sense. We then later sat down with Marcus and tried as best as we could to explain about the letter M and the golden arches. He seemed to understand and he finally did call a M, a M. He did love to eat at McDonald's, but he always got chicken nuggets. He would not eat beef, and so he would not eat a hamburger. He didn't began eating hamburgers until he was about ten or eleven years old.

*****

Marc's love for books continued and when he was three years old his favorite book was the Wizard of Oz. He had a book that had the cassette tape which went along with it and he memorized the whole book. He took the book wherever we went and he would pretend to read. People would stop and ask me if he could read. I was really tempted to say yes, but I'd tell them the truth, that Marcus had memorized the book. They were still impressed.

When Marcus was about three and a half years old, he decided he wanted to have characters to hold so he could act out the story. Since he couldn't draw, I would draw the characters and we would color them. Then I'd cut them out and put them on cardboard and add a popsicle stick to make puppets for Marcus to use to act out the Wizard of Oz.

I am not an artist. I just did the best that I could do. He would stand beside me and say thank you, over and over again. He was so happy that I was making the puppets for him. He loved my drawings. Bless his heart. He didn't know how bad they were. Marcus spent hours play acting.

It wasn't long until he discovered Superman and the Teenage Mutant Ninja Turtles. He was never Marcus in those days. He was always a fictional character. If I called him Marcus, he would say, "I'm not Marcus, I'm Superman," or whoever he happened to be that day. He also played by himself a lot. He would be in the middle of his play acting and did not like being interrupted.

Larry's parents, the Wilson's, loved to keep Marc. He was never any trouble. They had four sons and were very experienced with boys. Larry's mom bought this little stuffed character that was red. It looked kind of like a star. I don't know what it was. Whenever they knew we were coming over, Grandma Georgie would hide the critter and when we got there, Marcus would try to find it. He loved that game and it was something that was just between Marc and his grandmother. They played it for a long time. I really felt comfortable leaving him with them. Marcus loved them so much and they spoiled him rotten. They never demanded anything from him and seem to accept his differences with love. I think it was nice to have a quiet child in the house.

As you read this you may think that Marcus was a normal child, but as he got older, strange things began to happen. Things I found were very odd. I seemed to be the only one to notice these peculiarities.

*****

Marcus was very sensitive on his toes and fingers. When I would have to cut his toenails or fingernails, I would have to be very gentle and sometimes it was a fight. I would always explain why I was doing it, and he would have to be still or I could cut him. Also Marcus did not like getting his hair cut. He would sit very still while his hair was being cut, but he hated it. Sometimes he would kind of jerk and we would tell the barber that he was very sensitive on his head. We would go to the same barber for years and she was as gentle as possible.

He didn't like to get dirty either, especially his hands. We bought Marc a sand box and filled it with buckets and trucks and boy toys and he did play in it some, but it wasn't his favorite thing to do. We also bought him a Dalmatian puppy, whom he named, "Toto". Wouldn't you know. This was his, "Wizard of Oz", days. He loved that dog. Marcus has a very special love for animals, especially cats. He can't stand to see any animal hurt, not even a skunk or an opossum.

He hated getting wet unless he was in the bathtub. If he got a drop of rain on his shirt, he took the shirt off. I had a hard time with this. I just couldn't understand why he behaved that way. Sometimes we would have to run to the house from the car in a downpour and the first thing Marc would do is take off his *barely wet clothes*. He did seem to enjoy bath time and playing in the water sprinkler if it wasn't too cold. I didn't understand the difference.

Loud noises really bothered him. If we went to a parade and the band walked by, Marcus would cover his ears and cry that it was too loud. I would look around and notice that none of the other children were acting that way. A lot of chaos and loud talking also bothered him. He was not comfortable with yelling and if I was angry and yelled at him, it would seem to confuse him and he would cover his ears and tell me it hurt his ears. Everybody yelled in my family when I was growing up. I guess I had gotten used to it. I learned early on, that he didn't like it and it seemed to literally hurt him.

If he was watching a television show, or reading a book, when he learned to read, he didn't want any noise and he is still that way today. Outside noises really bother him when he is trying to concentrate. He doesn't want anyone in the room talking when he is watching a TV show or reading. (He could never be a mother, I can watch," Days of our Lives", talk on the phone, wash a load of clothes and cook supper all at the same time. Sometimes I read a book and watch television at the same time. Ha!)

He does not like being interrupted while in the middle of something, such as a book, movie, video game, or just listening to music. When he is talking, he gets very upset if he is interrupted. I guess a lot of people are that way, but in my family everybody talks at once and nobody listens to anybody. I have three sisters and my poor daddy had to live in a house of five women. He's so much like Marc and I do believe we drove him crazy. My daddy is very much at home with his chickens and goats. He loves books and stays in his room a lot, reading. He loves animals and kids and I believe Marcus has a lot of his characteristics.

    All of these things began to add up and I got the feeling that something was really wrong. Everyone that I expressed my concerns to, would tell me that I was just imagining things, even his doctor. My daddy told me all Marc needed was a good fishing trip. I was so frustrated. I needed answers. I guess because I was with Marc everyday all day, I noticed things that other people didn't. Marcus was very clumsy and uncoordinated. His fine motor skills were poor. He had a lot of trouble coloring in the lines and cutting with scissors. He was very apprehensive about trying new things and seemed stressed sometimes.

Chapter 3
Preschool

I began working at a daycare when Marcus was three. I felt that he needed to be with other kids, and if I was working there, then he wouldn't feel abandoned. I worked with the babies mostly, but I could see Marcus during the day. His teacher told me that he had trouble playing with the other children and seemed to be withdrawn. She tried to include him in the activities, but he wanted to play alone. I talked with her a lot and expressed my concerns. Marion was young, but she seemed to really care and wanted to help and she was the first person who noticed that Marcus was different from the other kids. He did enjoy the playground, but balked at the slide. Marion was very gentle with him and finally got him to slide, but he didn't get on it without help and a lot of coaxing.

I worked at the daycare for about a year and in that year, he never really tried to make a friend. He was happy playing alone or with Marion. He became very attached to her and looked forward to seeing her each day.

That summer Marcus began taking swimming lessons and he was having a very hard time. He was afraid to put his face under the water. All of the other children seem to be having so much fun, but Marc was not enjoying it. I was concerned because I wanted him to learn to swim. I wanted him to be comfortable around water. The first year of swimming lessons was not a success, but it was a start.

Marcus wanted a baby sister and I began to want a baby also after working with the babies at the daycare. Finally, Marcus got his wish when he was four and a half years old, Megan was born on December 30, 1986.

While I was in the hospital, Marcus had scarlet fever. He was very ill and was staying with his grandparents, the Wilson's. Marcus was terrified of shots. There was a nurse that worked at the doctor's office that was always very rough with the children. I had instructed the doctor that the nurse was never to treat Marcus ever again because she was so rough. My in-laws didn't know who she was and that day when I was in the hospital, *that nurse* gave Marc a penicillin shot. My mother in-law told me that the nurse stabbed him so hard, that he was bruised and he bled through his underwear and pants. Larry's parents are very loving people and they were extremely upset by the treatment of their grandson. I was in the hospital for eight days. When I was able, I called the doctor and told him what had happened. The nurse was fired. Mine was not the only complaint against her.

*****

A baby sister was a good addition to our family. Marcus really loved her. We had a lot of fun playing with her together. I think Marcus thought Megan was another stuffed animal until she got a little bigger. Right before Megan was born, I quit my job, so we had a lot of time to play. Marcus was very loving and gentle. When Megan got a little older he began including her in his acting. When she sat in her walker or little seat, Marcus would play with her and pretend she was one of his characters. She loved his animation. She was such a good baby and Marcus loved her. When I was pregnant Marc said he wanted a sister and if the baby was a boy, he would, "strow" him in the trash. I guess it's a good thing she was a girl.

Larry and I tried to play ball with Marcus many times again, but all he wanted to do was act, watch his TV shows, and listen while I read to him. He was very attentive.

By this time Marcus had Ninja Turtle, Superman, and Batman costumes. He was pretty much a happy child. I knew what would upset him, so I would try to keep the peace. He could get frustrated really easily if things weren't going right. If he couldn't find a particular book or a toy that he wanted, he would get upset and I would have to go help look through his book drawer or toy box until we found it. We kept all of his toys organized so they were easy to find and was less frustrating when looking for a particular toy. He had just about all of the Super Hero action figures that were made. He played all day pretending to be someone else. When Megan got old enough to actually play with him, he was on cloud nine. She was his April O'Neal or Cat Woman or Super Girl. They played well together. It was so funny. We had some old earphones that were huge and she would put them on her small head to be April O'Neal. She and Marcus would reenact the shows. Marcus finally had a playmate. This was when he began collecting the Ninja Turtle action figures and the super hero figures. Larry's mom and dad bought many super hero figures for Marcus to play with at their house. Each figure came with a small comic book and he just loved these. I think this is what began Marc's love for comic's.

Chapter 4
School Days

When Marcus was five years old he started kindergarten. Since he turned five years old on August 4th, he was a young kindergartner. Marcus had a lot of trouble with his motor skills, particularly his fine motor skills. His drawings looked more like a younger child and he still could not color in the lines. To try and cut with a pair of scissors was difficult. His balance was poor and he had poor coordination. He was a good boy, but he just had a lot of problems. His teachers loved him and said that he was very bright. They just couldn't read anything that he wrote. They would give him oral tests instead of written.

The actor really came out in him. He was so excited when the class began practicing the Christmas play. He was still shy, but he loved it. He has always wanted to be an actor. He was so shy that the teachers didn't realize his acting ability and this went on all through his school years.

Marcus had a lot of trouble making friends. The playground was still a problem and he also had P.E. to deal with. I guess he did his best, but he did not enjoy it. The P.E. teacher was a very manly woman and I don't think she liked Marcus very much. He was probably a sissy to her, but he did all right and survived. The kids laughed at him. He was very awkward and self conscious. He played alone each day and walked around the playground, playacting, never getting on the playground equipment. Around the first of school, Marc's class left the playground and he was unaware that they had gone back to class. When he played, he was in his own little world and was not aware of what went on around him. When he did become aware that his class was gone he became afraid and began to cry. Another teacher took him back to class and he got into trouble for not coming in when they did. He was only five years old. The teacher should have made sure that she had everyone before going back in. Actually his teacher, Mrs. Matthews was a very wonderful person. I will always love her. She was so good and kind to Marcus. I expressed my concerns to her several times and she agreed that there was definitely something odd about him, but she thought he was just young and would outgrow it.

Marcus told us something really funny about kindergarten when he got older. He said that Mrs. Matthews passed out M&Ms to the class and he thought they were Skittles. When he put one in his mouth and realized that it was chocolate, he spit it out and put it under the rug. We got a good laugh out of that.

Marcus began wetting his pants at school. He had never had any trouble in this area before. He was very easy to potty train and never wet his pants. The restroom was between his class and another class. *I mean it was right there*. Mrs. Matthews said that she always let the kids go when they asked. Marc told us whenever he felt the need to go, by the time he got there it was too late. We took him to the hospital where they ran numerous test, some which were painful and they couldn't find anything wrong with him. After that, the problem stopped. Mrs. Matthews sent him to the restroom often.

Marcus began having a lot of serious sinus infections and was still having ear infections. We had to change doctors because we changed insurance companies. I hated that because I loved his pediatrician. Some mothers at school told me about a wonderful doctor at the Scott and White Clinic. Marcus had a bad ear infection and so I made an appointment and took him to the doctor. I was surprised to find that the doctor was a woman. I was sure that I was told the doctor was a man. This woman was very rude. When she tried to look into Marc's ear, he pulled away. She was so mean. She told him that if he didn't sit still and let her look that she would get a nurse in there to hold him down. I was shocked. I told her that I would hold him, but she wouldn't let me. I couldn't believe it. I was young and naive. Now, I would have told her what I thought of her and reported the incident. When I took him back to school and told his teacher what had happened, she laughed and said I took him to the wrong doctor. That was Dr. B.'s *wife. She* specialized in treating kids with ADD and other problems. Of all people this doctor should have been patient and understanding. She should have picked up on Marc's problems right away. After all Ms. B. was trained in this area. She was supposed to be an expert in this field. Later, I took Marcus and Megan to her husband, Dr. B., and he was great just like everyone said.

Despite all of the problems, Marcus loved school and did very well. At the end of kindergarten, Marc's teachers wanted to keep him back another year. They tried to talk the school board into starting a Pre-First class, but they wouldn't do it. They finally decided to, the next year when it was too late for Marc. The teachers talked to us about how immature that Marcus was and felt that he could catch up if he had another year of kindergarten. We decided to let him stay back. It was the best decision that we could have made. He did very well the second year and because he was young, he didn't realize that he had been held back. His drawings were still poor and his writing wasn't legible, but no one could tell us what was wrong. He still had all of the P.E. and recess problems. None of that had changed. I also noticed he still didn't have friends and I tried so hard to help him make friends. Every birthday we would have a party and invite the boys, but it didn't work. He was not invited to their parties and no one played with him at school. His teacher was Mrs. Klement the second year and she was also a wonderful person. She was good to Marc, but she still didn't know what to make of him. No one did.

Each summer Marcus would continue his swimming lessons, but he made very little progress. He finally could dog paddle across the pool, but he would not put his head under the water and would not jump off the diving board.

Something else that Marcus did really bothered me. When he was watching TV, it was like he was in a trance. He was in his own little world. I would have to call him several times and sometimes go over and touch him to get his attention. He also did this if he was reading or even playing. I just thought it must be a man thing, and I was always telling him to come back down to earth.

*****

Both of the summers after Kindergarten, Marcus played T-Ball. It was hilarious fun. We had the best time. Once Marc ran around the bases after he was *out* and would not stop until he ran all the way to home plate. When he played out-field, he daydreamed and picked flowers. If the ball happen to come out to him, he would walk over to it and slowly pick it up and then walk back to the in-field and give it to someone, never getting in a hurry. One game he played hind catcher. Now in T-Ball, all the hind catcher had to do was catch the ball if someone was running for home and tag the person out. Marcus would not even attempt to catch the ball. He was afraid of it, so he would let it hit the fence, then he would go get it and walk right up to the umpire, standing about a foot away and throw it right at him. It was so funny. The umpire would say, "Now hand it to me," and every time Marcus would chunk it. It was great, but that was the end of his baseball career.

    We are Southern Baptist and Marcus grew up in church his whole life. When he was six years old, he expressed the need to become a Christian. In the Baptist Church, when a person has made a profession of faith and asked Jesus Christ into their hearts, we follow that decision with baptism. This means getting into a pool of water, (now there is a baptistry in the church building) and the pastor dunks the person under the water. This symbolizes the washing away of an old sinful life and rising up into a new life in Christ. Marcus wanted to do this, but he was so afraid of the water. He was not yet comfortable putting his head under water. We talked to the pastor about this and all agreed that we should wait until Marcus was sure and would not be afraid.

Chapter 5
First Grade

First grade was very different than his last two years. He was seven years old and older than most of his classmates. The symptoms he was having became worse and I was really concerned. Sometimes he just seemed to zone out and I would still have to touch him to bring him back to earth. Sometimes he seemed to be living in a world all his very own. At the beginning of the school year, I had a talk with the teacher and told her some of the problems that he was having. She did not recognize any of the symptoms. I told her how he would just day dream and how I would have to get his attention. Apparently she wasn't listening because when I went in to get him from school each day, she would complain that he wasn't listening. Well, I *had* told her. Finally, I stopped going in and I would just pick him up in the car line.

Marcus did well in first grade despite the problems. He became obsessed with drawing. He loved Winnie the Pooh and it was the first full book he drew. We bought him a big Winnie the Pooh story book. He still had a lot of difficulty writing and sometimes he would just draw the pictures and not finish the words. This was the beginning of a long journey of drawing and then writing books. At first he just copied the words and pictures in the books, then he began making up his own. He spent hours doing this and did not want to be disturbed. He went from Winnie the Pooh to Ninja Turtles. At first the turtle drawings were very funny, but gradually he began to get better. He wanted them perfect, just like the drawings in the color books and comics. Marcus began collecting the Ninja Turtle comics and enjoyed reading them and then making his own. Each day the children would draw a picture in a journal. Marc's pictures were so funny. I have kept all of his drawings and we have gone back and looked at his pictures and laughed until tears were running down my cheeks. He drew a picture of his teacher. It was a picture of a boy holding weapons and she wrote, " This is not my best picture, Marcus."

Marcus showed a good aptitude for math. His math teacher once complained that he was counting on his fingers and I said, "What's wrong with that, I still count on my fingers." Marcus showed more interest in plays and programs. That didn't surprise us, as he had been acting for years. He wasn't popular, but he had more friends that were girls than boys. This disturbed him, because he didn't want to play with the girls. Somehow he knew that would be weird, so he just played alone. He always said the girls were nicer to him than the boys.

Our family was always so protective of him. Everybody loves him. He can be himself with family and I know this is probably what has helped him the most. We have always given him so much support. Marc has been a family favorite in both families. He is very lovable.

Every night starting with kindergarten, we had school. Larry or I would sit down with him and do homework. In his younger years there wasn't much to do, but as he got older, he had more work.

Something happened that spring when Marc was in first grade and I think we could have lost him. Our church had a children's choir and the kid's were scheduled to go to Fort Worth to sing in a festival. I noticed the day before that Marcus' little finger looked as though he had been bitten by something and his skin was peeling off. We put medicine on it and kept an eye on it. That night before we were to go to the festival, Marcus broke out in a rash all over his abdomen. He wasn't feeling well and I wasn't sure that he was going to get to go to the festival. He had been so excited about going. I hated to disappoint him. The next morning he still had the rash, but he said he felt better. His finger looked worse. I was worried, but against my better judgment, we went. When we got there, Marcus began feeling worse and I really became concerned. The kids were wearing blue jeans and matching t-shirts. The day warmed up quickly and Marcus became very agitated and over heated. The rash had spread to his arms and legs. He became so upset that he didn't even get to sing. The ride home was miserable. The lady who was driving us offered to take him to the hospital, but I didn't want to put anyone out and Larry was at his parent's house with Megan. I just wanted to get him home.

As soon as we got back I called Larry and took Marcus to the emergency room, since it was a Saturday the clinic was not open. I had been giving Marc, Benadryl, but it hadn't helped. The doctor in the emergency room gave him something a little stronger and sent him home and said if it didn't go away by Monday to take Marc to his pediatrician. We waited until Monday and he was getting worse. We were so worried. I got him in to see Dr. B. (the wonderful doctor) and he immediately said he needed to take a blood test. He was very concerned. After the dramatics of getting blood, it was immediately tested and Marcus had some rare something (I can't remember the name). Dr. B. was concerned that it could have ruptured his spleen. I didn't understand any of it. I told him about Marc's finger and he looked at it, but didn't think that the two were related. He gave Marcus some strong medicine and he began to get well. We had to go back for several visits to make sure that he was okay. His finger finally healed. Larry and I thought that he had been bit by a brown recluse spider. We read up on the symptoms and it sure did sound like that. I guess we'll never know.

*****

The summer after first grade Marcus got a bike for his birthday. He was scared to even get on it at first. His balance was so poor that he had trouble riding even with the training wheels. After many attempts, he finally learned to ride, but would not try without the training wheels. He rode like this for several weeks and I began to think that he would never learn to ride on his own. Whenever we would suggest taking off the training wheels, Marcus would get upset and say that he didn't want to learn. Finally he allowed Larry to take the training wheels off, but Marcus still could not hold his balance long enough to ride and after a few tumbles he all but gave up. One day Teresa, my sister and Luke came over. Luke was so agile and athletic. He couldn't believe that Marc was still using training wheels. He took a few spins up and down the street and told Marcus that he would teach him to ride. Luke made it look so easy. It worried me some, but I kept and eye on them. A little while later Marc came running in and said he could ride. He was so excited. Teresa and I went out to watch. Luke was so proud that he had taught Marcus to ride the bike.

Marcus also began another round of swimming lessons. It just wasn't happening. He was afraid of water and the swimming lessons were probably a waste of money. All of the other children seemed to be doing well, but Marc would sink. We didn't think that he would ever learn to swim.

Being outdoors was not his thing. He couldn't stand to be barefoot in the grass. He wanted shoes on his feet at all times when he was out of bed. Also socks drove him crazy. He couldn't ever get the seam on the toe fixed to his satisfaction. This was a struggle everyday when he would get dressed. He absolutely hated sandals and I quit buying them. Summer passed all too quickly and school started again.

Chapter 6
2nd Grade and Discovery

Marcus started second grade, and his first day was lousy. There was a child named Philip that had appointed himself the torturer of Marcus. The first day, he was sitting across from Marc. The front of the desks were pushed together so Philip and Marcus faced each other. As they were getting settled, Philip grabbed Marc's school supplies and would not give them back. Marcus would get frustrated very easily, and he began to scuffle and argue with Philip. Mrs. Williams, the teacher, did not stop to find out what was going on. She just had them put their names on the board. Marcus was so upset when I picked him up. *This became a pattern that lasted many years.* I told Marcus, the next day, if Philip grabbed his supplies again, not to fight for them, but just sit there and look at him and see what he does. I told him if Philip would not give them back, that I would buy him more. I thought the child might be poor and needed the supplies.

The next day the same thing happened. Marcus did what I told him to do, and Philip got mad and threw them on the floor. Marcus said he bent over and picked them up and that was that.

Philip, *the child of Satan*, also sat by Marcus at lunch. This was a big mistake.

Mrs. Williams began calling me a couple a times a week, asking me to bring Marc dry clothes. Apparently, Philip had *accidentally* spilled juice or milk in Marc's lap. This began happening a lot. I discussed this with the teacher, and asked if perhaps it might be a good idea for someone else to sit by Marcus during lunch, but she replied that she had a seating order and didn't want to change it. When the behavior continued, Larry thought it was time to intervene. One day Larry decided to go and eat lunch with Marcus, and he just happened to sit between Marc and the child of Satan. Now, I'm not saying that he threatened the kid, but he very nicely suggested that it might not be in his best interest to spill anything else. It never happened again.

Second grade went down hill from there. Everyday at recess Marcus was still playing alone. He was still behaving very strange and would not play with the other students. Most of the boys were very rowdy and played rough. Marcus didn't like to play rough and did not like being touched or hit. He would not get on the playground equipment and did not enjoy playing ball. Each day he would walk around the perimeter of the playground and talk to himself. He also did this at home. The only difference was, at home was that he always had a weapon in his hand of some sort. Usually it was a stick, sword, or play gun. At school sometimes he would pick up a stick or rock off of the ground. Needless to say, he had no friends and was very troubled about this. He just couldn't understand why the other boys wouldn't play with him. Many days when I picked him up, he would burst out in tears and tell me about his very frustrating day.

*****

Marcus was not happy and I talked to his teacher about it often. This was only her second year to teach and she was as baffled as I was. Each night we would have school all over again and do his homework. He said that he could not concentrate in the classroom with the noise. I wanted Marc to be the best that he could be, with as little stress as possible. I noticed that he was having trouble copying from the book to the paper. It took him a long time. I began dictating to him and he not only learned the material, but his homework went a lot faster.

Second grade drug by and the year was finally coming to an end. Academically Marcus was doing great, but socially it was awful and he was very unhappy. He cried a lot and asked me several times why the other kids didn't like him and why was he so different. At church he was basically ignored by the adults. Megan was so cute and outgoing. She never met a stranger and could carry on a conversation when she was very young. I have to admit that she was quite adorable. Marcus would come home crying sometimes and ask me why they loved her, but didn't love him. I tried to explain to him that people always liked little girls because they are so cute, pink and frilly. It made me angry that adults can sometimes be so without a clue. I tried to calm his feelings and assure him that he was loved by everyone, but I really didn't know what to do. Then one day we got answers.

Mrs. Williams had really become concerned and I guess she wanted to know as much as I did, what was wrong with Marc. One day the OT (occupational therapist) came to the school to work with the students who had physical disabilities. Marc was not in Special Education and therefore not eligible for services. Mrs. Williams asked Ms. P.(the OT) to watch Marc on the playground for a few minutes and see what she thought about him. She watched him and told Mrs. Williams that she was pretty sure that she knew what Marcus had. When I came to pick him up, his teacher was so excited and wanted me to talk to the OT. She said that Ms. P. thought she knew what was wrong with Marcus. I couldn't believe it. After all of this time someone was finally going to put a name to what was wrong.

I met with Ms. P. and she said that she would like to test Marcus on her own time. She couldn't legally do it through the school, because he was not in Special Education.

After school she tested him. Her evaluation told her exactly what she had thought. Marcus had Sensory Integration Dysfunction (S I Dysfunction). I had never heard of this and she suggested that I take him to Scott and White Hospital and have him tested again and there he would be able to get services. Mrs. Williams knew who to call and she set up the appointment for us.

At Scott and White Hospital, we met Karen Wylie, an OT. She was very good with Marcus and she retested him and came up with the same answer. It really was a relief, even though it was scary, to finally know that Marcus did have something wrong and it had a name. Then I could say to everyone, "I told you so." It was not a spiteful thing, but I was so tired of people telling me that I was just imagining things. (According to Carol Stock Kranowitz, M.A. a Short definition for Sensory Integration Dysfunction is the inability to process information received through the senses. I found this in her book, (**The Out-Of-Sinc Child.**) I found this book a couple of years ago at a book store while looking for another book. I was so surprised when I began to read it. I was reading all about Marcus. I wish that I had of read this book when he was younger. It could have really been enlightening and helpful and I would not have felt so helpless.

Marcus was in occupational therapy for almost a year, thanks to the *Children's Miracle Network*. They paid for everything that he needed. Larry was employed full-time at the First Baptist Church and we had no health insurance at the time. Karen was so great with him. She knew just what he needed and she provided it. We were always included in every aspect of his therapy and she explained in detail what was wrong and what we could do at home to help. His fine motor skills were very poor. While in therapy Karen helped Marcus make a trivet for my kitchen. It is heart shaped, using different shaped tiles in the mosaic style. They put mortar in between the tiles. I will always cherish it. It represents the suffering and trials Marcus went through and the love we have for each other. The tectile thing was big. He didn't like to be touched. We would put him on a blanket and pull him around the house. Megan got in on the excitement. It was a fun time. I also would rub his arms with a soft towel and put lotion on his arms and legs. He wasn't too comfortable with the lotion. We were still having trouble cutting the fingernails and toenails, but Marcus always suffered through it. At Scott and White, Karen took Marcus into a room that had a container filled with crushed corncobs. The corncobs were warmed and Marcus would put his hand into the warmed corncob mixture and feel around for toys hidden inside. He seemed to really enjoy this activity after he got used to it.

There were many activities for Marcus at Scott and White. He seemed to be getting a little better. One thing I remember that he did was lay in a tire swing on his belly and as he would swing, he would pick up bean bags and throw them into a bin. He also rolled around on a big ball that was on a mat of course in case he fell off. Karen always was so good with Marcus. She was kind and loving and very understanding when he was afraid. She never gave up on him and we will always be grateful to her for all she did. Now that Marcus is twenty two years old, I can still call Karen and talk to her about Marcus and tell her of his miraculous improvements. All of the one on one attention helped his self-esteem, which was very low. He always felt inadequate. Marcus began seeing a child psychologist to talk about his feelings.

Mrs. Williams was so happy to finally help Marcus, that she began working with him on the playground. She would try to involve the other children. The girls were mostly the ones who wanted to help, I guess they had that mother instinct. The boys didn't seem interested. At that time Marcus couldn't walk a balance beam or swing and wouldn't slide. The equipment was very high and just too scary. I remember there was a little girl named Annie and one day when I came to pick up Marc, she ran up to me with a big smile and said that she had taught Marcus to swing. The girls were playing mother hen, but the boys still ignored him and it hurt his feelings.

When school was out, Marcus continued the therapy twice a week. We also continued swimming lessons, which still were not working. It was embarrassing for Marcus. All of the other children were jumping off the diving board and swimming to the side of the pool. Marcus finally did it, his daddy had to get in the pool with him and catch him. I think he bribed him with a new toy. Marcus was terrified and wasn't excited about repeating the process. Megan was taking lessons in the beginners class and she was

out swimming Marcus. That was so humiliating for him. Megan was doing so good at swimming that we stopped the lessons. We decided to invest in a small above the ground pool. It was only about three to four feet deep, but it was great for dog paddling. Megan was swimming up a storm. I think it gave Marcus the incentive to learn. We practiced all summer and at the end of that summer Marcus was swimming. He wasn't as afraid because it wasn't over his head. We also began going to the city pool more and he did eventually learn to swim better. Now, he loves to go swimming. He's not that strong of a swimmer, but he jumps off the high diving board and does great.

Marcus was also becoming quite an artist. Drawing was taking up a lot of his time. He was getting better every day. His fine motor skills were also getting stronger. He had a lot more coordination. I think all the hours that he spent drawing really helped him. He became so good that a local restaurant put one of his pictures up on the wall.

By the end of the summer, life seemed to be looking up. His therapy was going well. Marcus was doing a lot of activities he never would have done before. We began playing ball. We bought this game that had two paddles with velcro on them. A tennis ball came with the game. All a person had to do was stick out the paddle and when the other person threw the ball, it would stick to the velcro. The game was called, "Scatch".

Marcus really liked this game. We then began looking for other games that would help his eye-hand coordination. We bought balls that would not hurt if he got hit and also bouncing balls. He could not bounce a ball very well. We worked with him daily. The therapy at the hospital and at home seemed to be helping his self esteem and coordination, but then as all good summers have to come to an end, this one did. Reality of the third grade occurred and it seemed all the good that we had accomplished in the summer was wiped out.

Chapter 7
Third Grade Woes

Marcus was looking forward to the third grade. We had a great summer and he felt he was ready. We weren't prepared.

I had a meeting with his new teacher a few days before school started. I told her all about Marcus and about SI Dysfunction. I told her about his low self-esteem and how he really had a hard time relating to the other students, especially the boys. I thought she understood. She seemed to be receptive to what I told her. We had known her for several years. We had gone to church with her some years before and I had always thought that she was a nice person. I could not have been more wrong. As Marcus looks back, he will tell you that she was one of the worst teachers that he ever had, if not *the* worst.

It just began with little things. She would be short with him, and Marcus would come home and tell us. She would say things like, "Marcus is not listening. I asked him to bring me a book and he brought me a pencil." Then she decided that he had ADD. I told her he did not have that, but she was convinced. She began to lose all patience with him and so did his math teacher. They would gang up on him and the poor child would be all upset when I picked him up. It started happening a lot.

We went to a doctor at Scott and White (not Dr. B.) We had to change doctors because he started only seeing patients with stomach and intestinal problems. We told the doctor that his teachers thought that Marcus had ADD. Without even testing him, he put Marcus on a drug called Cylert. It was horrible. Marcus stopped eating and lost interest in everything. He began having awful nightmares about demons and monsters. He would wake up in the middle of the night, screaming. He couldn't sleep. We called the doctor after a week and told him what was happening and he said not to give him anymore of the pills. Finally, we decided to have him tested for ADD so his teachers would be satisfied.

We took Marcus to the child psychologist that he was already seeing at the time at S&W Hospital. Marc was so unhappy and the doctor told us that if we would bring him to the clinic and leave him, they would test him for ADD. He was tested for almost five hours. They discovered that he *did not* have ADD. He had a normal IQ and had scored extremely high on the tests. They also said he sat through all the tests and loved it. He was not hyper at all. They were impressed with his behavior. Marcus had always loved one on one attention and he usually got along well with adults. It was his peers that he always had trouble with.

We took the results back to the school and I think it made the teachers mad. They did not agree with the doctor. I then requested that Marcus be tested for the gifted and talented program and he did well and was put into GT. I talked to the school counselor (Nancy Mercer) and she was wonderful. I requested that she check in with Marcus once in a while because he was so depressed and so she met with him once a week. I told her how unhappy that he was and she was great. He felt very special when he was with her and loved all the attention.

Marc's two teachers were still having problems with him. I personally feel that they just didn't like him. There are two things that happened that year that we will never forget. Marc's homeroom teacher, Ms. T., told the students to get their books and go to math. They did change classes in the third grade. Marcus was sometimes slow about getting things done. He probably wasn't listening and realized that they were leaving and began to look for his math book and assignment. Ms. T. yelled at him to, *"Just go"* and he told us that he tried to tell her that he didn't have his stuff, but she wouldn't listen. So he reluctantly went to math class unprepared. When he got in math, Ms. R. asked him where his math book and homework was. He said it was in his desk. Marcus said that he tried to tell her that Ms. T. wouldn't let him get it, but she just told Marc to put his name on the board and go back to his homeroom and get his things. When he got to his class Ms. T. yelled at him, "Why are you back in here?" He told her that Ms. R. told him to get his math. Now, by this time both classes were laughing at him and he was crying. He got his things and went to math. When I picked him up that afternoon, he was still crying. He told me what had happened and I was very upset. I wanted to cry *for* him. You must understand, Marcus was a very sweet and loving child. I have worked in schools for fifteen years and we do not treat our children like that. When we told Larry what had happened, I must say he lost it there for a little bit. When he calmed down, the next day Larry went to the school and had a long talk with Ms. T. I'm not exactly sure what he said, but I'm sure it wasn't pleasant. After that day we didn't have any more trouble from her that I recall. She still was not friendly, but I never heard of any more episodes. Karen Wiley offered to come to the school and talk to his teachers, but everything seemed to get better.

The other thing that happened, really made me angry. Marcus was required to learn all of his multiplication facts from one to twelve. He was in an accelerated math class. The only acceptable grade was a one hundred for his multiplication facts. We worked and worked with Marcus every night through tears and frustration, but he did learn them. Ms. R. gave each child several chances to make the one hundred. She promised the students an ice-cream party at the end, for everyone who completed all the tests with a one hundred. The day before the party, I thought about the fact that Marcus did not eat chocolate and I wanted to make sure that she had some vanilla ice-cream. I called her and asked what kind of ice-cream they would be having. She was very unfriendly and responded that she had bought Eskimo Pies for each child and they would be sitting outside on the curb to eat them. I told her that Marcus did not like chocolate and she said, "Well too bad." If I wanted him to have something else, I would need to buy it and bring it to the school for him. Marcus had been looking forward to this *party* for weeks. I don't call sitting out on the curb and eating an Eskimo Pie, a party, but I didn't say anything about it to Marcus. The next day I brought Marc a orange push-up pop. It was fine and he never knew that I was upset.

Marc decided that he was finally ready to become a Christian and was willing to be baptized. Our pastor at that time, Dr. Mark Bumpus had talked with Marc and assured him that he would not let him drown. Larry took

Marcus into the baptistery, minus the water, and described the process. Marcus wanted to be baptized on Easter Sunday. On March 31, 1991, Marcus was baptized at the First Baptist Church of Troy, Texas.

*****

He began making whole books with the pictures and illustrations. Most of the books were *The Teenage Mutant Ninja Turtles* (TMNT) at first, but then he began making up his own comics. I remember one of the books was *Water Man*. He was still collecting comics and if he wasn't drawing, he was reading. He has several collections of comics by this time. He also started drawing *Sonic the Hedgehog*.

Eventually third grade ended and we were all glad for that. Marcus hated third grade. He did however make a friend. His name was Zeb, and Marcus finally had someone to play with. His therapy ended at S&W and we had a good summer. We practiced on swimming and playing ball, constantly working on Marc's motor skills. He was still having trouble with my cutting his toenails and fingernails, but things seemed to be getting better everyday. I had learned to be more patient and understanding with him.

Chapter 8
Fourth Grade

The elementary school that housed Pre-k through third grade was too crowded for fourth grade and so the fourth graders were moved to the Intermediate and Jr. High school campus. The fourth graders had their own building on the other side of the campus. The lunchroom was also in this building. The students had to walk across a gravel parking lot to go to P.E. There was no supervision to and from the gym. The teacher was a coach, which was a bad idea. He was very abusive to the students who were not athletically inclined. One day in P.E. the students were complaining about doing exercises. Marcus was humming while he exercised. Coach D. (a very overweight, unattractive man) called Marc to the front of the class and told him since he liked to sing, to come up and sing "Mary Had a Little Lamb" and then he would let the boys go out and play football. He then told the boys to clap for Marcus. Coach D. then *made* Marc go to the front of the class and sing. He was so humiliated. The boys were laughing and making, "Baa, Baa", noises. We had always taught Marc to be respectful to the teachers and to mind them, so he sang while they all laughed at him. Marcus does not enjoy playing or watching football, therefore he didn't do it so they could go out and play. He did it because he was intimidated by the coach. That day he cried the whole class period. The boys laughed and made fun of him all during class and made fun of him as they walked back to their building. When he got back to class, his teachers saw how upset he was. They took him to the teacher's lounge to try and find out what had happened to him. Marcus was very fortunate that year. He had two wonderful, loving teachers, Mrs. Dworsky and Mrs. Mayo. They really loved Marcus. I guess it helped that they both went to our church and I had kept them informed of Marc's progress. They already knew about the SI Dysfunction. Marcus was so upset, it took a while for them to understand what had happened to him. When he finally told them what had happened, they were furious. I was substituting at the high school that day and Larry was working at the First Baptist Church. Mrs. Dworsky told me what had happened and I called Larry and he went to the school. The teachers also called the principle, Mrs. Smith over and they had a little meeting.

    The next day Larry and Mrs. Smith went to the P.E. class. The coach never apologized or gave an excuse for his behavior. After that Marcus had a new name for the coach. He called him Coach Doughnut Hole. His name was similar to that and Marcus just changed it a little. The man was very overweight. He could not have run around the track if he had to, yet he harassed the students all year long. Something that I have learned is that *most* coaches do not like kids who are uncoordinated or not athletic. They have very little tolerance for these kids. Marcus' worst class was always P.E.

    I began to notice that Marcus was becoming very nervous. He started tapping his pencil on his desk a lot. Mrs. Mayo told me that Marc was getting on her nerves, but she laughed about it. She said he was a very good student. He always did his homework and did well on tests. Each evening we were still having school at home. Larry and I helped Marcus with his homework and we helped him study for tests. He learned how to study and has therefore done well with his class work. Megan is a very bright kid, but I feel we have always done her a disservice by not giving her the attention that we gave Marc. She is so independent and strong willed. She has always wanted to do everything herself. Even when she was two years old, everything was, "I do it myself". Marcus just required more attention and help. Megan is his opposite. She is beautiful, very outgoing and never meets a stranger. She loves everybody.

    One day Marcus told me that he couldn't copy all of the notes for science from the overhead. I just thought he was slow at copying because his trouble with eye tracking. He copied the notes from a sweet little girl in his class and it became the norm. It never occurred to me that he might have trouble seeing.

    Marc's class took a field trip to Salado (a small tourist town south of where we lived) and then went to a park for a picnic. Somewhere by the park there were men cutting down trees. The wind was blowing very hard and a piece of sawdust blew into Marc's eye. He told the teachers, but he said that he was pretty much ignored. They couldn't do anything about it, after all they had a lot of other kids to watch. He suffered all afternoon and when we went to pick him up from school his eye was in bad shape. His teacher came out and apologized and said that she didn't realize that it was that bad. We called the doctor when we got home and the nurse said to put a wet cloth on it and wait and see if it got better, but it didn't. We waited too long and ended up having to take him to the emergency room. We were in there three hours. Marcus had a big chunk of wood stuck in his eyeball under his eyelid. They had trouble getting it out. They put a suction cup-like thing on his eye and flushed it out with water. His eye was very irritated. He was so tired and upset. Every doctor's visit seemed to be traumatic for him. It's no wonder he hates doctors and hospitals.

*****

Marcus played basketball with the "Little Dribblers". For those of you who don't know what that is, they divide the students up and play basketball games against each other. It gives the younger kids experience in playing basketball before they enter Jr. High school. It is not mandatory, and it's supposed to be just for fun. Some of the parents took it a little too seriously. We were supposed to be teaching our children good sportsmanship. Some of our parents never learned that when they were kids. They would yell and scream at the kids and it was disgraceful. Marcus tried his best and had a good time. That's all we wanted. High school students were the coaches and they did a far better job I think, than the adult coaches would have done. They were kind to all the players no matter how good or bad they were. Marcus played Little Dribblers for two years.

*****

While Marc was in fourth grade and Megan was in Kindergarten, there were afternoon cartoons on the Fox station. During and between cartoons the station invited kids to be on the show. They had little spots in which they would tell about upcoming events and they would ask the kids questions. Marc and Megan applied and were invited to be on the show. It was around Halloween. They taped a full week of shows in one afternoon and played one segment each afternoon. M&M were both so excited. They so wanted to be discovered.

The summer before fifth grade Marcus and Megan made a tape to be sent to the Barney Show. They were both very talented (all parents think so). We went over to the church and made a tape of them singing and talking. Megan has always been a talented singer since she began talking. Marcus wanted to act so bad that he made the tape hoping a talent scout would discover him and he would become a famous actor. We sent the tape, but we never heard from them. Marcus' dream has always been to act. He does have talent, but he was shy and felt he wasn't good enough. Even his teachers really never gave him a chance to prove himself.

*****

That summer Marcus had the opportunity to go to Pre-Teen camp with the children from church. Any child who had completed 4th through 6th grade was invited to go. He was so excited. I think deep down, he couldn't wait to grow up and get away from so many problems. Pre-Teen sounded so grownup to him. Megan loved to aggravate Marc whenever she had the chance. When he said that he was going to camp, I think Megan was a little jealous. She began pestering him. She would tell him, "You are not a teenager." Marcus would get so frustrated and say, "I'm a Pre-Teen." That was an ongoing argument that summer. Megan got the biggest kick out of tormenting him. Marcus was so proud to be a *Pre-Teen*. He said that word many times that summer. Megan thought it was so funny. She took every opportunity to get him to say it just so she could laugh. It did become kind of comical after a while. We all got a good laugh about it later.

Chapter 9
Fifth Grade

Marcus had four different teachers for fifth grade. His homeroom teacher was his science teacher, Ms.B. We had known her for a long time. Living in a small town you know just about everyone. I again went to her and talked to her about SI Dysfunction. When Marc was in school only a few weeks, Ms. B. happened to mention that the teachers had all gotten together and had a little meeting with Marcus. Needless to say we knew nothing about the meeting. I was very upset when she told me that they had a meeting with Marcus and didn't let us know that they were having a problem. Ms. B. said that Marcus was not participating in class. He never volunteered answers and they felt that he needed to participate more. I asked her if he was disrupting the class and she said," No." I asked if he was turning in his homework and she said, "Yes." Really there didn't seem to be a problem at all. She did admit that Marcus was in tears when the meeting was over. I was so angry. I couldn't understand why they had the meeting at all. Marc's social studies teacher told me that she was against the meeting and told them so, but they still went ahead with it. I talked with the principle and she knew nothing of the meeting. I really liked Ms. Smith. She was always so supportive. I felt that I could trust her. She talked to the teachers and she assured me that nothing like that would happen again. Marc's social studies teacher told me that Marcus was her favorite student. After that happened everything went smooth. I explained to the teachers the reason that Marcus never volunteered answers is because he was so afraid of being laughed at. The boys treated him badly and he was intimidated. He had been humiliated before and just wanted to go to school and do his thing with as little notice as possible.

Marcus always did very well in math. One day he came home and had a math paper for me to sign. He had made a "3" on the paper. Yes, you heard me right, out of a "100", he made a "3". I about died laughing. I couldn't believe he make such a low grade. He said he copied the problems off of the board and I guess he copied them wrong. I should have gotten a clue about his eyesight, but I didn't.

There was still the problem with P.E. Coach Doughnut Hole had left, but there was still no supervision from class to P.E. One day on the way to the gym Marcus was teasing a new student about a girl. I guess he became a little braver or he felt comfortable teasing the student because he was new. I don't know, but he was teasing him and the student became angry and punched Marcus in the stomach. Marcus said he spun around like a Ninja Turtle and kicked the boy in the head. (Showing off his acting skills?) About that time one of the coaches came out of the gym and saw only that part. Ms. Smith called me and told me what happened. I went up to the school and talked to her. I told her Marc was wrong for teasing the boy, and she agreed, but she said Marc was only defending himself when the boy hit him. There was a school rule about fighting, so the other boy got two days in ISS (in school suspension), and Marcus got one day. I cried all day and when I went to pick him up, he had a smile on his face. He had thoroughly enjoyed his day. Nobody bothered him. He got all of his homework done, finished his library book and he didn't have to go to the dreaded P.E. class. Marcus also got in trouble at home for the fighting and teasing. I don't remember now what his punishment was, but we had a long talk about teasing. I wanted him to remember what it was like to be teased. It really upset me because he had been through so much and I wanted him to learn from it.

There was a boy who was athletic, good looking, and very popular. The problem was, he was bullying the other boys in the locker room. He was harassing the other boys who were unpopular and throwing people up against the wall. It apparently became a regular thing. I didn't complain because it didn't happen to Marcus as far as I knew. He would come home several times a week and tell us things that happened in the locker room. I did mention to the principle one day that it would be a good idea for the coaches to keep an eye on the boys, but they told her that they didn't go in the locker room because they could be accused of doing something wrong. They told Ms. Smith that they stood outside the door and listened and never heard anything going on. Marcus said that they never stood outside the door. That year this particular boy was awarded with a citizenship award. It was unbelievable.

Marcus continued to have trouble socially. He had his ups and downs. Some days seemed to go fine and some days ended in tears. About this time Marc started liking girls. He wasn't popular and his self-esteem was low. Whenever he liked a girl, she always had a boyfriend. Fifth grade ended without incident.

*****

Summer was always met with excitement. No homework and all the free time in the world. Marcus and Megan always looked forward to vacations and family reunions. Summer was a great time.

On a trip to the grocery store we discovered that the child was blind. We were sitting in the car while Larry went in the grocery store to get something. A girl walked across the parking lot with something written on her shirt. I told Marcus to read her shirt. He couldn't see the girl and Megan read the shirt. (Naturally, Miss Priss) A red flag went up. I then asked Marcus to read the license plate on the car in front of us. He couldn't read it either. I really became concerned. On the way home, he tried to read the road signs. He couldn't read any of them, not even the big green signs that hang in the middle of the interstate highway. The next day I called the school and asked the secretary for his eye test results from fifth grade. It was very bad. Marcus couldn't see. Then I understood why he had trouble copying from the overhead or the chalk board. He couldn't see it. The part time nurse we had at the school didn't call to let me know that Marc needed glasses. No wonder he had made a "3" on his math paper. It all made sense after that.

We took him to the optometrist and he got new glasses. I couldn't believe his face when we walked outside. He had never seen clouds before. He was so amazed at what he saw. The roofs on houses looked so different. He thought the shingles were one big piece. He didn't know they were separate.

The leaves on the trees had been just a big blur. He could finally read signs. I asked him why he didn't tell me that he couldn't see and he said he that didn't know. He thought everyone's vision was like that. So far the SI Dysfunction had affected every one of his senses. Some kids have more severe symptoms.

*****

Gradually his fine motor skills had gotten better. By now he had a Nintendo game and he and Larry played often. It really helped his eye hand coordination. He was still drawing regularly and that was helping his fine motor skills. His coordination and balance was somewhat better. In fifth grade he even began playing the trumpet in the school band. That was hard for me to believe since he hated loud noises, but he loved it. Things were really changing. He still would not eat chocolate or ketchup. To this day there are still things that he will not eat, but he does have a big variety of foods he likes. He finally began eating beef and pork. After a while he even began eating hamburgers. I never thought he would. He loves steak and pork chops now. Things began to look up.

*****

Fifth grade ended and once again we had a great summer. We lived in the church parsonage since Larry was the music minister at the church. The pastor was buying another house. Across the street was a boy in the grade ahead of Marcus. They were about the same age because Justin only went to kindergarten once. Justin had a basketball goal in his driveway. He invited Marcus to come over and play with him. Marc really enjoyed those days. Justin was popular in his class and it made Marcus feel good to play with him. They became good friends. They also played video games together. It was really good for Marcus. I will always count this family among my best of friends. The whole family was wonderful to us. Eddie and Nita always stood by us. They have a daughter, Rebecca, one year younger than Megan. They played together a lot. Angela their oldest child, was several years older than Justin, but we loved her too. When Eddie was mowing his yard, many times he would just drive across the street and mow ours. There are wonderful people in this world. Now that we no longer live there, I miss Nita a lot.

*****

Larry began building us a new house in the country the summer of 1994. Since Larry has had a carpentry background and has helped in building several homes including his parents home, he decided he could build ours. He did a great job. It took him almost a year, working only on Saturdays and sometimes on his day off during the week. He had a lot of help from his father and some help from friends. The summer of 1995 we moved in and it was great.

Chapter 10
Sixth Grade

Marcus was really beginning to have a great sense of humor. We laughed often and we discovered that he had a talent for comedy. He decided to become the class clown. Instead of the kids laughing at him, they would laugh with him. I'm not sure he got the response he wanted. We can really be a silly family and we have always wanted our children to have a sense of humor. Larry and Marcus both can imitate people on TV. Marcus is very good at imitating cartoon characters. He sounds just like them. I think it is so sad that kids are not taught to get to know a person before they decide they don't like them. We as humans are too ready to judge people on appearance. If someone is labeled a nerd or geek, they really have a hard time living it down.

I think Marcus was learning to enjoy school. He wasn't coming home upset quite as much and he was laughing more and having funny stories to tell. He still had social issues, but he was growing up and learning to cope. I'm sure I babied him too much, but I just wanted everything to be perfect for him and you can't make everything perfect.

We discovered that one the boys that Marcus had befriended was actually his cousin. My mother went the funeral of her cousin. When she got home she called me and told me that my second cousin lived in our town. I knew the family well. We were friends, but I didn't know that we were related. Marcus thought that was pretty cool. His friendship with the boy was up and down. Just the way with kids. One day they were friends and the next day they were not. I think that since Marc had a reputation of being the class outcast most of his life, some of the boys who would ordinarily have been his friend, would not, for fear of being labeled odd. Everyone has the need to be included in the group. It really hurt Marcus to be ignored and excluded from any group at all. He needed to feel accepted by someone. It was very hard for him.

There was a bright light in Marc's life that year. It was his math teacher, Ms. Mosley. When she spoke to the children, she would say," Now Ms. Mosley doesn't like that", or "Ms. Mosley is watching you". Marcus thought she was hilarious. He always came home with funny stories about *Ms. Mosley*. She spoke with a very country accent and he had fun imitating her.

Chapter 11
Seventh Grade

Marcus was very happy to finally be in Jr. High school. He felt so grown up. His exceptional math skills were becoming apparent. He did well in all of his subjects. Marcus began seeing the counselor (Elizabeth Geiger) with his social problems. She was always very understanding and helpful. I felt comfortable talking with her.

*****

I remember that Marcus had an assignment to write about John F. Kennedy for social studies. He wrote that, "He was a good president and a good father, but he had lots of women." We really got a good laugh out of that.

Teachers reading this need to watch the way that you behave around kids. They pick up on everything. Marcus came home and told me that his reading teacher and his science teacher really liked each other. He told me that they always stood out in the hall and talked. I told him that they were married to other people and were just working friends. Marcus said, "No, mom, you don't understand. *They really like each other*." Several years later after we had moved away, I found out that they really did like each other and were in fact divorcing to be together. Kids are so observant. Be careful what you do and say.

*****

That year Marcus was given a special national math award. He was nominated by his math teacher that he adored. He was also a very good reader. I guess reading all those comics was paying off. He got to read Jurassic Park and he loved that. They also read a book about flour babies. They had to carry around with them all day a baby made of a five pound sack of flour. If the sack was damaged it would affect their grade. We dressed Marc's flour baby up and put it in a small basket. I remember Marc took it to school with a small bear in the basket. Someone stole the bear. Marcus was so upset about that.

After the book was read and the assignment was over Marcus and Larry took the flour baby out and used it for target practice. It was great. Marcus laughed and laughed.

*****

Marcus also began playing Jr. High basketball. He was on the B team and he felt that he was better than that, but he still enjoyed playing. The coach didn't let him play often, but when he did, he loved it. I think it was just being included in a group that helped his self-esteem. We loved going to the games and watching him play. It was just like T-ball all over again. It was fun.

*****

After two years of playing the trumpet, Marcus was getting pretty good. He loved it. Music was always a big part of our lives. He still wasn't sure what type of music he liked, but he listened to all kinds. He got a kick out of his band teacher. Marcus said when his teacher would call his name Marcus would respond, "Huh" and the teacher would say, " Don't grunt at me." Marcus thought it was funny and the kids would laugh. Finally he was getting some positive feed back from the other kids. He learned if he acted up, and got in trouble, then he was finally fitting in. The kids laughed with him, not at him. It kind of became a joke between him and the band director. We were out shopping one day and we went in a store that made special t-shirts. We came across an iron on sticker that said, believe it or not, "Huh". We got that shirt and Marcus couldn't wait to go back to school so he could wear it. He went to band and when the band director called his name, Marcus proudly stood up and pointed to the word, Huh. The teacher made him go stand out in the hall, but he said it was all worth it because the kids all laughed and cheered. He came home that day very excited. He was indeed learning to be the class clown. He wasn't a typical class clown though, because he took his school work seriously and still was an a honor roll student. There was a lot of smart kids in his class and a lot of competition.

Marcus was still having some trouble with his coordination and balance and peer group, but it seemed to be getting better. Seventh grade ended pretty much the way it started. Marcus seemed to be a lot happier most of the time.

Chapter 12
8th Grade

Marcus began the school year with great anticipation. He was a good student. If his peers had of been more accepting of him, I think it would have been better.

He really was seriously getting into video games and the more he played, the less he read and drew. He lost interest in drawing altogether and I was sad to see that. Technology began taking over everyone's lives. He became very good at video games. It was a challenge to see how long it would take to win the game. We all played with him sometimes, but he was so good, I didn't have a chance. Megan played some games with him, but most of the games were not very interesting to her. By now she was in the fourth grade and was as cute as a button. Everyone loved her. She was becoming an outstanding singer, taking piano lessons and was popular with her peers. She had many friends, unlike her brother. Between homework and outside activities, she didn't have lot of time to play with Marcus. When Larry wasn't at home I was elected to play video games with him and I'm terrible, but Marcus was always encouraging and loving. He didn't care how bad I was, he just needed a playmate even if it was his mother. We have always had a very special bond.

He was still doing well in his classes despite his lack of social skills. His teachers loved him and always were very complimentary of him. It had been this way for most of his school years, excluding third grade. He was really a great kid and could have proved that if he had been given a chance. I think he just finally stopped complaining about his social problems. We tried to teach him to be proud of himself. We tried to teach both of our kids to be honest, loving and trustworthy. This old world is a hard place to live. People are taught to be judgmental and critical and it is up to the parents and teachers to change that way of thinking.

Marcus did pretty well in the eight grade. There were some things that would never change with this set of students. Marcus was the way he was going to be and that wasn't going to change either. We had come to realize that life was pretty much the way it was going to be and we had learned to accept it and take each moment as it came.

Then things changed. A music minister search committee came to our church searching for a new associate pastor. They came to hear Larry. Apparently they liked what they saw and heard, because they wanted him to come to the First Baptist Church of Hillsboro. This would mean a big change for all of us. We prayed about this long and hard. We wanted to be sure that it was the right thing for our family.

The school year was coming to a close and we weren't sure what we were to do. I think we were waiting for God to give us an answer. I was by this time working at the high school full time as an aide. Megan was flourishing with her music. Larry enjoyed his job at the church. Then I believe God gave us his answer. Larry went to pick up Marcus from school that last week. He came out crying and had little cuts all over him. Three boys had ganged up on him in the locker room and threw him into a full length mirror, which broke into many pieces and cut Marc. Larry went in the gym to try and get answers from the coaches. They said they weren't sure what had happened, but they would investigate the incident. I called the principle to try and get some answers, but he was not helpful at all and never had been, since Marcus had been in Jr. High. He said he was leaving the incident and punishment, where appropriate, up to the coaches. I felt that was just a cop out on his part.

Since the boys who did this to Marcus were popular boys, absolutely nothing happened to them. Marc said the coaches tried to get him to say that it was his fault and that he had provoked the attack. Marcus told us that the boys were harassing him and making fun of him and he took up for himself. That's when they pushed him into the mirror. The coaches decided that all the boys were at fault including Marcus and made them do extra exercises in P.E. That was it. Once again the unjust are justified and the victim is victimized. This is a sad world.

We decided to go to Hillsboro in view of a call. We needed to get Marcus away from these boys. The church voted to have Larry come as their new associate pastor. Marcus was not the only reason that we decided to move, but he was a big part of our decision. We truly felt God was leading us in this direction.

It was a very hard decision for Larry. We had only lived in our new house for two years. Larry had sweat and bled over that house and spent a year of his life building it and it was very difficult giving it up. Megan was not happy. She had many friends and her music was going well. She was having to give up a lot. She really was not given a choice. We voted as a family and she lost. Marcus was so excited about moving. He had been tortured by these kids for so long, he just couldn't wait to get away from that school and make a new start.

I found out later that after we moved, the kids found other students to pick on. They didn't have Marcus to push around anymore. The principle once again would not get involved and the parents of the unfortunate boys went before the school board. The principle eventually left. I'm not sure what the circumstances were. I do know that it was his responsibility to take up for the kids who were being persecuted and he did not do his job. Since we were no longer there, it wasn't Marc's problem anymore. We put those days behind us and looked to the future.

We moved to Hillsboro in the summer of 1997. Even though it was scary to move, it was also kind of exciting. I was going to miss my friends. We told each other that it was not that far away, but we did end up losing touch. I hate that because good friends are very hard to find. We do still talk sometime on the phone and ever great once in awhile we get to see our old friends, but not often enough.

Chapter 13
Starting Over

Larry began his new job and felt somewhat overwhelmed with so many new responsibilities. He was not only the music minister, but the educational director and church administrator. For those of you who don't have a clue what I'm talking about, let's just say it was an enormous job. I got a job at the elementary school working as the fine arts aide. Megan was beginning fifth grade and Marcus was beginning high school.

That summer the kids worked hard to get acquainted with the school kids at church. I was disappointed to find out that there were no kids at our church Marc's age. It seemed hopeless sometimes. He really needed to make friends before school started.

The church had a lot of activities for the youth, but Marcus was still shy and uncomfortable around strangers. It seemed the only people that he was comfortable around was family. We all loved and accepted him just the way he was.

He decided what kind of music he liked and to my shock and dismay it was metal music. Actually I really don't call that stuff musical, but I guess everyone has their own opinion. He wanted us to buy these CDs. We were so much against this type of *music*.

We really wanted Marc to listen to good uplifting, musical, music. I listened to a lot of Christian music, but I also enjoy many country singers. Whenever I complained about the music that Marc chose, he would comment that country music was not always wholesome and he was completely right, but the music I like usually has good lyrics. He really began to get enthralled with these bands. We absolutely refused to let him listen to death metal, but we did allow bands whose lyrics weren't that bad. The singers had horrible voices. They were very unpleasant to listen to. It was more like screaming or growling than singing. I think Marcus was just trying to find somewhere that he could fit in.

Chapter 14
Ninth Grade

Marcus has always been timid and afraid to do anything new and unfamiliar to him. Larry took him to school since the church was only a few blocks away. We watched him struggle to find his place. I hoped and prayed that he would find friends, not just any friends though, good Christian friends. The first few weeks seemed to go smooth. We went to church and school and that was about it. I missed the friends we left behind. It was a lonely place to be. We all were having to start over. It was difficult.

Megan began making friends, but even for her it was hard. The music teacher that I worked with, realized that she had an exceptional talent and there was some jealousy with the other girls. We began working on," Grease" the musical, and there wasn't a lot of talent to choose from. There was another girl in Megan's class who has a very good voice and she and Megan sang several of the lead girl's songs. They both did very well. When Megan sang, she got a standing ovation. It was great, but Megan was once again getting all the attention. Marcus needed to find his niche.

He enrolled in band and journalism and all the other required classes. I really wished that he would take some art classes, but he seemed to have lost interest.

Marcus had done very well in Algebra I in the eighth grade. He made all A's, but there was a required exam that he had to take. He has never done well on these type of tests. When he took the exam, he was told that it didn't matter if he passed or not. In his old school he would still be passing Algebra

I and go to the next math class in high school, which would normally be geometry. This all happened before he knew we were moving.

He did not pass the exam. He made a 68, I think, which was not passing.

We learned in Hillsboro that a student must have passed that exam to move on and since Marcus didn't pass, he would have to repeat Algebra I. Even though he made all A's in the class in eighth grade, it didn't matter to them, so he began repeating the class.

This school had a strange schedule. Each class that would normally be a whole year class and one credit, was taken all in one semester. The classes were longer and there was more homework, but at Christmas break, the class was finished. A student could take more classes at this rate and get more credits. I kind of liked this schedule, but I didn't have to do the work.

This meant that Marcus had two chapters of Algebra to do each night. It was a lot to do. After about three weeks of school and a lot of math problems, a meeting was called. Apparently most of the kids were behind and already failing the class. Marcus was not one of them. He was keeping up and doing well. He even told us that he was helping the other students in the class. The teacher didn't actually teach the class. The students were given a schedule at the beginning of the year and each week they were given a test over the homework that they had done. After doing the homework, hopefully each night, they would go over it in class each day and if a student didn't understand the work then the teacher would go around and help those who didn't understand. This is where there was a problem. The one teacher could not possibly get around to all of the students who were confused. He also did not grade the homework. It was supposed to only be to help a student understand it enough to pass the test. Each student who actually did their homework got a "100" each day whether the work was done correctly or not. This in my opinion is no way to teach. Marcus and a few other students who understood the lessons ended up helping the teacher tutor.

At the meeting it was discussed that the kids were failing, the class was too large and the teacher could not help that many people by himself. I didn't even understand all of it at the time. I never heard anyone say anything about the teacher not really teaching the course or grading the papers. Larry asked the question, "If the teacher did not have time to give *individual attention* to each student, then how were they going to pass?"

I guess the question was taken the wrong way because, the next day they pulled Marcus out of the class and put him in Social Studies as well as a couple of other students. While talking to the counselor, she said, since he needed *"individual attention"* that maybe he should be pulled from the class. He came home very upset. Larry had to go to the school and straighten it all out. Marcus was doing very well in the class and Larry told them that Marcus *would stay* in Algebra I and finish the course. I don't know what they thought they were doing by pulling him from the class. The teacher even told them that Marcus was helping tutor some of the other students. Marc was then left in the class and at the end of the year actually had the highest grade in the class and received a math award.

The English class was pretty tough. It was an honors class and there was a lot of required reading. Marcus had pretty much lost interest in reading, and was not thrilled in the assignments. There was a big difference from Jr. High and High school. The classes were a lot harder.

Marcus enjoyed marching band and loved the teacher. He did have some difficulty marching. It does take a lot of coordination and balance. I remember watching him march the first few football games. It was really quite comical. After a few performances, he began to get the hang of it. It was his favorite class. Since he was in the band, he did not have to take the dreaded P.E. That was a relief. Since this was a larger school, there were more boys who didn't take athletics.

We were very involved in church and Marc had the youth group who did things together often. He still did not feel included that much. Since there were no boys his age at the church I think he still felt left out. Even in church there are little clicks and we have never been a part of that kind of thing. It even happens with adults. That's probably where their kids get it. I believe Marcus began to feel kind of turned off by church. That has been hard for me to accept, but he will have to make his own way in this world.

*****

In ninth grade Marcus began taking driver's education. I worried that he would have trouble driving or be afraid to drive, but he did quite well. He really enjoyed it. We had moved to the country by this time. We were twelve miles from Hillsboro and it was a good road to practice driving skills on. Larry began letting Marcus drive to school in his car and I would go pick he and Megan up and let Marcus drive my car home. It gave him a lot of practice. We continued to attend church and go to school and work. Marcus was still not making friends and that really concerned us. Megan was even having trouble finding her place. It is so hard to fit in when you move to a new town. The kids who have lived in the town their whole life tend to stick together and they don't like new people joining in. It seems there is so much competition for your place in a group.

 Marcus finished ninth grade and seemed to have done well. Megan was going to sixth grade and had proved to be a very talented and outgoing young lady. The summer before tenth grade Marcus got his driver's license. We bought him a small car. He was so proud of it. He was really growing up before our eyes.

Chapter 15
Tenth-Twelfth Grade

I realized that Marcus was still not over his SI Dysfunction. He only drove to the school and church. He would not detour anywhere else. He would not get gas or go to a restaurant or get his haircut. He wanted his father or I to go with him. I tried to tell him what to do, but anything new scared him. Larry went with him to get gas and made him put it in the car and go in and pay for it. After a few times, he was finally comfortable doing it. He always worried about going over on the pump and not having enough money to pay for it. I told him to always plan on getting less than the money that he had in his pocket. That way if he went over a little bit, he would still have enough money to pay. Far a long time Marc would not go by himself to get a haircut. I would give him the money and he would call Larry to meet him there. Finally he began doing this on his own. He would not go to a restaurant by himself. I don't know why that was, but I think when he went with friends a few times, he got more comfortable. Yes, he eventually began to make some friends and the younger kids at church were kind to him. Everything with Marcus has been baby steps, but he is getting there.

Marcus' skills on the trumpet were getting better every day. He still loved band and felt a special bond with the teacher. As he got older, the marching became easier. He seemed to be outgrowing many of the problems that he had when he was younger. I notice he still has a problem with the touching and he does not enjoy playing rough. He gives great hugs and I know he is comfortable with his family.

I was still cutting his fingernails and toenails and one day I just told him that he was going to have to learn to do this himself. I had to be very patient, but firm. I told him I can't be going off to college with him and cutting his nails. He learned and keeps them cut nice and short.

He also began having to shave. He was not thrilled with this, but soon got the hang of it and resolved to the fact that he has to shave. It just keeps growing back. Now he still waits about a week before he shaves. When it starts itching he gives in.

*****

On the way home from school one day Marcus had a wreck. In order to get to our house, one must turn left at the blinking yellow light in our small town. There was a teenager driving rather fast and he wasn't paying attention. When Marcus began turning, the driver from the other car started passing him and ran right into the driver's side of Marc's car. It totaled the car. I was also coming home from work and when I got close to the intersection, I saw there had been a wreck. I then realized that it was Marc's car in the wreck. I pulled over and ran to the car. Marcus wasn't in the front seat and I was imagining awful things. I began asking the teenagers from the other car where my son was. They just looked at me. Then, to my relief, Marcus came out of the store across the street. He had gone in to call his daddy. The other car was full of teenagers. I think one girl broke her wrist. None of them were wearing their seatbelts. The DPS arrived and the driver was given a ticket. His father's insurance company paid for the damages. I don't know if the boy was on his insurance or not, but the man didn't even question who was at fault. The lady working in the store, said those kids came by the store everyday just flying. She said she knew that one day there was going to be a wreck. Marcus did hit his head on the steering wheel, luckily he had on his seatbelt. He just had a little scratch where his glasses were. It really shook him up. He was a little scared to drive after that, but we got him another car and he eventually began driving again.

His junior year he asked a girl to the prom that went to our church. She agreed to go with him, but as soon as they got there, he said she left him and went to be with her friends. They didn't even dance. He was very disappointed that it turned out the way it did. He only liked her for a friend, but she was rude to him.

The end of his junior year he got a job. He really surprised me, that he did so well. He was growing up before our eyes. He had a few problems because he had never worked with the public before. Taking checks and credit cards and counting out cash took a little getting used to. His job was working at KB Toys in the Outlet Mall in the town. He waited on customers, unloaded trucks and stocked the shelves. He also had to price the toys and clean the store after closing. He really liked this job. The longer he worked there, the more comfortable he became. His boss, Ms. Brooks was a Godsend. She was wonderful with him and was like another mother. He loved working with her. Several times he was invited to her home for Super Bowl parties. They treated him like one of the family.

His senior year went by pretty good. He began making a few friends. He was inducted into the National Honor Society at the end of his junior year and band was going well. He had been taking "Theater" for four years and it was his favorite class. He could be himself there. His teacher, Ms. Simpson, (his favorite teacher) let him be himself and she loved him. They had so much fun in that class. They did many skits and lip singing. Marcus came home often and had tales to tell about what happened in that class. That and band was his highlights of the day.

Marcus also loved mythology. He loved all the stories about Zeus and he loved the plays by Shakespeare. Literature was one of his favorite subjects. At the end of the year he took a friend to the prom. They had fun. Mollie is such a sweet girl and she and Marcus get along so well. This prom turned out a lot better. His senior year ended good.

He graduated sixteenth in his class. He had done very well. There were eighty-five graduates. Marcus made the decision to go to Hill College, a junior college in Hillsboro. He wanted to still live at home and continue working at KB Toys. He wasn't sure what to major in and so he just majored in Liberal Arts for the time being. He enrolled in band and really enjoyed his time playing the trumpet. He did very well academically, but after two years at that college Marcus had still not made many friends. He had a couple of friends from high school and a couple from KB's. There were many acquaintances, but not any lifelong friendships. I think the main problem that

I can see now that he has grown up, is his lack of social skills. I think he feels awkward around strangers and doesn't really know how to react around people that he has just met.

Marcus finished Hill college with many honors and received his Associates Degree in Liberal Arts.

Chapter 16
The University of Texas in Arlington
Moving out!

For the first time in his life Marcus was moving away from home and living on his own. He was so excited. I was worried. My baby that I had spent so much time with was no longer going to be around. I was pretty much a basket case. Marcus was very optimistic. There was a mix-up at Hill College and Marc's records didn't get sent to UTA in time and the dorms filled quickly. By the time that we were able to get registered and mistakes from Hill college corrected, there were no dorms left. Marcus was going to have to live in an apartment. There were apartments right by the college that only housed college students from UTA. We went through all the steps required to move in. It was still difficult to get everything done that was required. We weren't sure who Marc's room mate would be. When he finally moved in, his room mate turned out to be a very nice guy and they got along well. During the second semester however, he was called home for a family emergency and Marcus finished out the year alone.

Marcus began marching band. The practices were very rigorous. He started a couple of weeks before school actually began. In Texas it is very hot in the summer. If you recall Marcus is not an outdoor person, but he survived. He even started getting a tan. The best thing was, he felt like one of the guys and felt like he was making friends.

His first semester he made a 4.0. He had decided to major in Art. Now

I know that it sounds strange, but we went over every major that UTA had to offer and every job known to man and he didn't find any of them appealing. Finally I decided that he would major in art. It was coming down to the wire and he had to declare a major.

After a few weeks of art he told me that he was enjoying his classes, but he thought that he was not talented enough. He was doing his best, but he was still having trouble with his fine motor skills. He was so nervous that his hands shook when trying to draw straight lines and the dreaded cutting with scissors. After two semesters of Art he decided that he would change his major to Business.

Chapter 17
Senior Year
UTA

His music likes have changed to Power Metal and it has become very important to him. This music is still metal music, but there is a lot of orchestra mixed in. He really enjoys concerts of his favorite music artists. The loudness doesn't really seem to bother him now, although, sometimes he wears earplugs.

His, *should have been senior year*, started out pretty well as a business major. Very soon he discovered that he did not like business. He hadn't had any math classes since his first year at Hill College and he had never taken Calculus. It was a required course for business majors. He knew very early that he wasn't going to do well in this class. So in the first few weeks of school he dropped his Calculus class and then changed his major to Broadcast Communications. After realizing that he had a lot of credits that didn't go with the new major, the second semester, he changed to Interdisciplinary studies.

This major was a conglomeration of many different subjects. It was still possible for Marcus to take his communication classes. He is now in his final year of college (hopefully!) and he is having a ball. Although he is having to go to school this summer to get all of his classes in, he is enjoying it. Last semester he had a radio show for one hour a week at the college. He really seemed to enjoy it. Now he is making commercials and editing them. I think he may have found something he loves. They are having so much fun. He has made friends. He has a great sense of humor and still seems to be doing well.

He has some friends who enjoy camping. Now I know I told you that he is not an outdoor person, but he is learning to enjoy the outdoors and I think it's good for him to toughen up. He swims often at the apartments and is getting a tan.

I truly believe that he is in for great things in his life. The Lord has blessed our family tremendously and I think all of Marc's problems has brought our family closer together. M&M are getting along so well now that they are growing up. They had the usual sibling rivalry. It was so hard for Marcus when Megan was so normal and outgoing and he was always in the background craving attention and not receiving it from people.

Megan has now graduated high school and is going to Dallas Baptist University in the Fall. She is doing well with her music. She is a beautiful young lady. She is leaving her cheerleading days behind and I know when football season rolls around each year, she will miss it a little, but she has so many things to look forward to. She is, (for now) majoring in communications, but her dream is music performance. Maybe someday, the Lord willing, she will make her dream a reality.

Both of our children are following their dreams and I want all of you to know that there is hope for all kids with problems and disabilities, with the love and compassion of parents and teachers.

I am still working at the elementary school that I have been at for eight years. I love the children, but I can spot those with characteristics like Marcus' rather quickly. I am more compassionate to these kids. I have shared the book, The Out-of-Sync Child, with the counselors. It is so important for the word to get out there about Sensory Integration Dysfunction. It is more talked about then it used to be, but there is still more that could be done. All teachers should be aware of it's affects on children and try to work with the child and parents with understanding and compassion. Marcus is going to be all right. He's on his way and I feel very confident that my "Out-of-Sinc Child" is getting "in sinc" with his life and it's all going to work out for the best. He is enjoying life and making new friends everyday. Lives so exciting for him. I pray that God will guide him in his endeavors and he will do great things.